# HOME REMEDY SECRETS TO OVERCOMING PREMATURE EJACULATION

**Rebecca Taylor**

# HOME REMEDY SECRETS TO OVERCOMING PREMATURE EJACULATION

# REBECCA TAYLOR

*Copyright © 2017*

*All rights reserved*

# TABLE OF CONTENTS

# INTRODUCTION

Premature ejaculation is one of the most widely talked about subject in the men's world. As it poses a significant problem to the masculine fold, most men who have the issue do not fancy talking about it with anyone, unless they get in contact with some trustworthy doctor or friend.

Truth be told, not everyone likes to blab about their sex life, or in this case, dysfunctions, with other people. The larger percentage of persons prefers to keep it a secret and stay out of discovery's way. Premature ejaculation, something very peculiar to men, is not in any way an unserious issue, as many have found themselves with the condition, and usually are oblivious of what led to it, what to do about it, and how to go about solving the problem.

Sadly, many men do not know they have the problem, as some of them remain sexually inactive until a certain period in their lives when they get in contact with the opposite sex, and the sudden realization that they don't last in bed throws them into phases of self-doubt and misery. Premature ejaculation, according to Wikipedia, occurs when a man experiences orgasm and expels semen soon after sexual activity and with minimal penile stimulation. In some genres, it is called early ejaculation or premature climax, usually, because it happens all too soon during sex, leaving the man disappointed and frustrated, and the woman unsatisfied.

There are no standard cut-off times for defining how long a man should last in bed, but a team of experts at the International Society for Sexual Medicine endorsed a definition including "ejaculation which always or nearly always occurs prior to or within about one minute. T

he International Classification of Diseases says that premature ejaculation usually occurs within 15 seconds or less after engaging in sexual intercourse.

To both sexes, premature ejaculation often causes distress. But particularly for men, it devastates and makes them crawl up into their shells, avoiding relationships due to shame and fear of being discovered. Overtly, the premature ejaculation problem affects more males than females, as the distress level in the latter is lesser, as most of them do not have issues concerning the men not being able to have a swell time with them.

However, some women do fall to distress due to under- satisfaction, not just nymphomaniacs but averagely sexually-active females too. Statistics show that one out of every ten men experiences difficulty in lasting longer in bed at some point in their life. It interferes substantially with the sexual pleasures of the man or his partner. When it occurs on a widespread footing, it becomes a medical problem.

Moreover, there are some claims that premature ejaculation is a psychological state of being, while some say its biological and others claim it is a distinctly medical state. In the United States, one out of every three men of 18 to 59 years old has problems with premature ejaculation. Also, some experts say that in every man's life, once or twice, despite the fact that he may be sexually healthy, he experiences premature ejaculation.

The second Ad Hoc International Society for Sexual Medicine (ISSM) Committee for the Definition of Premature Ejaculation defined acquired premature ejaculation as a male sexual dysfunction characterized by the development of a clinically significant and bothersome reduction in ejaculation latency time in men with previous normal ejaculatory experiences, often about 3 minutes or less, the inability to delay ejaculation on all or nearly all vaginal penetrations, and the presence of negative personal consequences, such as distress, bother, frustration and /or the avoidance of sexual intimacy. In some cases of the literature, it is called an erectile dysfunction or a sexual performance anxiety prostatitis.

In the psychological approach, consensus about the definition of premature ejaculation has never been reached due to conflicting ideas about the essence of the syndrome (Marcel Waldinger).

Waldinger goes further to say that Masters and Johnson and Kaplan suggested qualitative descriptions, i.e., female partner satisfaction or man's voluntary control. Masters and Johnson defined premature ejaculation as the man's inability to inhibit ejaculation long enough to satisfy his partner 50% of the time.

Waldinger says that this definition regarding a partner's response is rather inadequate since it implies that any male who is unable to satisfy his partner 50% of sexual situations could be labeled a premature ejaculator and since it would also imply that females "should" be satisfied on 50% of the intercourse.

Waldinger went further in positing that another way to define premature ejaculation is by using quantitative measures such as the duration latency, or the number of thrusts prior to ejaculation. Definitions according to the length of time prior to ejaculation, varied from 1-7 minutes after vaginal intromission.

Waldinger says that these cut-off points were not derived by objective measurements, but were subjectively chosen by the various authors. Premature ejaculation according to him, was a matter of (many) minutes, and men who ejaculated within seconds were qualified as severe cases, and that equally subjective cut-off points have been proposed for the number of thrusts as a criterion for premature ejaculation: ejaculation within 8-15 thrusts.

The central nervous system controls ejaculation. When men are having sexual intercourse and are stimulated, there are a number of signals sent to the brain and spinal cord. All men do not have the same levels of excitement, and as such as do not all have the same ejaculatory brain signal system. When a man reaches his level of excitement, signals are sent from the brain to the reproductive organs.

These signals trigger hormones and other bodily chemical compounds, causing semen to be released through the penis. The sperm moves from the testicles to the prostate and mixes with seminal fluid to make semen. To expel the semen, the muscles of the base of the penis contract when orgasm has been reached. It is, therefore, safe to say that usually, orgasm and ejaculation occur at the same time.

However, some men have been found to reach the peak of sexual excitement without ejaculating. Sometimes, an erectile dysfunction may be the cause of premature ejaculation, being a case of a man not being able to get or keep an erection that is firm enough for sex. Usually, the erection goes away after ejaculation, making it hard to know if it is a case of pure erectile dysfunction or premature ejaculation or a compendium of both

. Due to this, most men are often thrown in a quagmire, unable to differentiate which from which, and identifying which one it is that bothers them.

According to Wikipedia, although men with premature ejaculation describe the feeling that they have less control over ejaculating, it is not clear if that is true, and many or most average men also report they wish they could last longer. General, after all is said and done about the horologic calculations, men's typical ejaculatory latency is approximately 4-8 minutes.

The opposite condition, in which men spend too much exhaustive time during sexual intercourse before ejaculating, is called delayed ejaculation. A biologist, Hong argued that premature ejaculation in men is nothing but an evolutionary adaption to enable men to pass on their genes quickly and rapidly.

Premature ejaculation should not be minced with pre-ejaculation. Pre-ejaculation involves the release of a less potent substance called pre-ejaculatory fluid, usually occurring due to intense sexual excitement before vaginal penetration. Pre-ejaculation is less of a problem than the troublesome premature ejaculation.

# CHAPTER ONE

## History of Premature Ejaculation

Premature ejaculation, like every other dysfunction in the human system is traced back to the position that male mammals ejaculate quickly during intercourse, cajoling some factions of biologists to posit that rapid ejaculation is an evolutionary condition that wafted its way into men's genetic makeup in order for the chances of passing on their genetic signatures to be increased.

The problem's control issues have been undergoing series of documentation for more than 2000 years. There was an Indian sex book in the 4th century called the Kamasutra that was widely read at the time. In it, it was said that generally, women love the men whose sexual energy lasted for a longer time, but they resented men whose energy expended quickly because he stops before they reach their climax and cuts them from their satisfaction. In some other vain, not all the intellectuals regarded premature ejaculation as such a problem.

Alfred Kinsey, a researcher, was one of such people. He viewed the condition as a sign of "masculine vigor" that could not always be cured. A thorough explanation for this opinion remains unavailable. According to Marcel D.

Waldinger, the history of premature ejaculation is a history of contrasting hypotheses, controversial debates among medical specialists and psychologists, many opinions, and ignorant and embarrassed patients, but it is also a history of independently thinking clinicians, and pioneering clinicians and neuroscientists, who all together and throughout the years contributed to a better insight in a syndrome that for a very long time has been neglected in medical sexology and general medicine.

This goes a long way to show that in one way or another, everyone and is involved in the development and explanation of the topic, and not just based on general principle, but the individual convictions of people.

Just as it has to do with the convictions of people, the history of premature ejaculation also have been influenced by groups of people. People from different parts (countries, to be specific) of the world have their own legacies to offer about the topic. Although the term "premature ejaculation was not invented until the 20th century, the condition remains as old as humanity itself. As far back as 2000 -3000BC in Egypt, the Egyptians celebrated sexual intercourse and every other if its entailment, or everything that goes with it.

As it was, there was a prescription for the male sexual dysfunction, and it was the lotus flowers. Men smelled the flowers and inhaled the scent which created a blissful feeling and in some ways helped in reducing anxiety, lessening the chances of premature ejaculation symptoms manifesting. In Israel and Judah, a very interesting account was recorded. In the book of Genesis, it was written that God hated the wasting of one's seed (semen).

Onan, after marrying his sister-in-law upon his brother's death, found that he could not orgasm inside his wife. Modern interpretations show that it meant that Onan did not have total control over his ejaculatory tendencies, hence, premature ejaculation. As a result, he spilled the semen on the ground, and God killed him for it because it displeased Him.

In India, between 400 BCE and 200 CE, there was an author, Mallanga who discussed in the book Kama Sutra, some men's tendency to ejaculate prematurely; "The first time of union, the passion of the man is intense, but on subsequent union, the reverse of this is true…if a male be long-timed, the female loves him the more, but if he be short-timed, she is dissatisfied with him.

China on their own part had their history with the topic. The Tang Dynasty as it was called, was a sexually liberal period in all of

Chinese history. Sex was seen and accepted as an endeavor that was good for one's health (which is still held as such till today). Nevertheless, the Chinese thought that ejaculating quickly weakened a warrior and depleted him of his chi.

So the Tang Chinese set to work and developed an intense behavioral training that will enable men to stop premature ejaculation and even reach orgasm without ejaculating at all. Lastly, Tunisians had their own orientation between 1500 -1600 CE. A Tunisian, Sheikh Nefzawi in his book on lovemaking and sexual health, "The Perfumed Garden" said that: 'When the mutual operation is performed, a lively combat ensues between the two actors who frolic and kiss and intertwine. Man in the pride of his strength works like a pestle, and the woman, with lascivious undulations, comes artfully to his aid. Soon all too early, the ejaculation occurs.

All these historical tracings go long ways to show that despite the seemingly recentness of the premature ejaculation topic, a lot has been in store regarding it, showing that it didn't begin all of a sudden today or yesterday, but that it has been since time and its antiquity.

# CHAPTER TWO

## Types of Premature Ejaculation

Ejaculation, as it has different ways in which it manifests, also has different types. Widely, a total of four types have been recognized and based on their differences, they are given special treatments, and countless debates have followed it as well. There are lifelong, acquired, subjective and variable premature ejaculation types.

## Lifelong Premature Ejaculation

Manu males have been found to have had the premature ejaculation problem for not just a while, but for the entirety of their lives. A lifelong premature ejaculation usually is found at when the male has his first sexual intercourse. A percentage of men with this anomaly inherit it from their fathers as the gene can be passed onto offspring if the problem is not checked and solved.

A series of research carried out by a neuropsychiatrist, Marcel D. Waldinger, have come together to show that 91% of lifelong premature ejaculation cases are caused by genetic factors, proving the aforementioned right. A patient with this type of premature ejaculation is likely to experience difficulties in solving the problem, but that does not translate to it being unsolvable. Several cases have been treated.

## Acquired Premature Ejaculation

This type often comes as a surprise, usually because of some causal factors. It is the condition in which a male who has had a healthy sex life from the onset and has recorded some levels of standard overall performance suddenly starts to experience premature ejaculation during sexual intercourse.

As earlier said, it is affected by factors, and examples are stress, anxiety, and depression, or fear that might be related to a fresh relationship, as well as seemingly unrelated issues such as work or finances. Many at times, it could be a result of poor dieting or malnourishment. Hormonal, serotonin and emotional or mental imbalance could be the causes of acquired premature ejaculation.

This type is easier to cure, as all that is needed to do is eliminate the factors that led to the development in the first place. Most times, as a result of it being caused by the man's temporary feelings, it could go away as the feelings elapse, returning the man to his usual performance level. In other more differential cases, some treatments will have to be conducted.

## Subjective Premature Ejaculation

This kind of ejaculation occurs based on thoughts and feeling. It is a condition in which a male thinks he experiences premature ejaculation, either on a consistent or inconsistent basis.

Upon being told by a doctor or a sex therapist that there is really no problem or cause for panic and worry, the male will still persistently believes that there is something wrong with the time it takes him to ejaculate, and as such will still go on in the search for a way or method to delay ejaculation further than he is currently able to. Subjective premature ejaculation is characterized by a male having a preoccupation with his imagined premature ejaculation or a preoccupation feeling as though he cannot control the timing of his ejaculation, leading to stirs of worry, panic, and depression.

This kind of premature ejaculation is mostly associated with younger adults who really do not have an insight of the cutoff time for ejaculation during sexual intercourse. This undoubtedly can be corrected with some orientation.

## Variable Premature Ejaculation

As the catchphrase 'variable' suggests, it is the type of premature ejaculation that occurs irregularly or inconsistently or on a random basis.

# CHAPTER THREE

## Causes of Premature Ejaculation

For a man to understand his seemingly embarrassing predicament, as to why it is beyond him to control himself and last longer in bed himself so he and his partner can enjoy sex, he first needs to know what the causes of premature ejaculation are. As is a popular saying, one cannot solve a problem without first getting to the root of it.

The source of premature ejaculation is tapped, having long protrusions that web their ways into each other and in different dimensions. What this is trying to say is that there are figuratively a millions causes of premature ejaculation. On the first ask, a layperson would tell you that the excessive intake of sugar by men is what causes them to ejaculate all too soon.

No doubt about the position being correct, but then, that's just generalizing. Not all cases are caused by diabetes mellitus, in fact, this does not in any substantial way measure up to half of a quarter of the causes of premature ejaculation.

Most men have been found flipping through endless pages of books and scrolling pages on the internet, looking for a cure, when in fact the way to cure something is to know what causes it.

Premature ejaculation is caused by several factors and these factors more detailed underlining causes.

**Physical Factors**

The physical nature of a man and his environment can cause premature ejaculation in a lot of ways. His physical health can determine whether or not he will last long in bed. And, when the physical cause of the problem is talked about, there is a very close relationship drawn with medicine.

This means that a physical condition can also be medical. There are many medical conditions which cause the problem. They include underactive thyroid, diabetes, high blood pressure, multiple sclerosis, prostate disease, urethritis, stress, excessive alcohol intake, drug abuse and laziness (although these are not medical but physical).

## Underactive Thyroid

This is also known as hypothyroidism. The condition is caused by the inability of what is called the thyroid gland to produce sufficient hormones such as thyroxin. This failure leads to a wide range of symptoms which may manifest in weight gain, depression, fatigue and a drop in libido, also known as the sex drive. The last three symptoms are primarily what lead to premature ejaculation, and particularly, the last. Fatigue will make the man's sexual organs not perform well, and they will not be able to respond well in order to delay ejaculation.

A drop in libido is the apogee of it, usually occurring when the man feels fatigued and depressed at the same time. He will lack the sex drive to penetrate the vagina and stay on long enough to strike the crescendo of sexual excitement. The man, with his systems nor functioning properly, and his sex drive inactive will ejaculate too quickly and then start to feel weak. Most men who suffer from underactive thyroid choose to remain sexually inactive until the medical condition is either suppressed or cured.

## Diabetes

Diabetes is a medical condition where there is excessive glucose or sugar in the bloodstream, and, as mentioned earlier, is caused by excessive sugar intake which inhibits insulin production in the digestive and circulatory system. Insulin is produced in the pancreatic duct (precisely in the islets of Langerhans), and it helps to break down glucose content in the blood to make it less lethal to the entire system. But where there is a case of shortage of insulin production, diabetes occurs. Sugar levels that are poorly managed cause damage to the autonomic nerves which control sexual arousal and this then affect blood flow and all kinds of sexual activity.

The outcome of the predicament is premature ejaculation, retrograde ejaculation (a case in which semen passes into the bladder instead of leaving through the penis) and an erectile dysfunction.

**High Blood Pressure**

Medically, this is termed hypertension. It is common in these modern times. Occurring due to pressure exerted on the walls of the artery as blood flows through them, it causes the heart to pump blood harder through those tight passages, increasing the risk of a heart attack or stroke.

The arteries that pump blood to the penis are not excluded from the pressure and the damage, meaning that the reduction in blood flows into the reproductive organ results in an inability to gain an erection, which then leads to premature ejaculation. The sperm cells do not receive enough blood to act normally and with the expected vigor.

**Multiple Sclerosis**

This disease occurs as result of the damage of the coating around the nerve fibers, called the myelin, which then inhibits the transmission of signals from the brain to the body. Muscle weakness, poor coordination, blurred vision, and muscle spasms are the likely symptoms that emerge.

These symptoms reduce the person's desire for sex, and this includes both genders. In men, there are fewer erections and the sensitivity of the cells around the penis is irregular. This makes sustaining an erection harder, leading to premature ejaculation.

**Prostate Disease**

Medically, thus is termed benign prostatic hyperplasia. It occurs when there is a sudden enlargement of the prostate gland. This increase exerts pressure on the urethra, impeding the flow of urine and semen down the tube and out of the body through the penis. In a larger sense, it makes the flow irregular; sometimes fast, sometimes slower. This creates an avenue for the unprecedented flow of semen to cause premature ejaculation.

**Urethritis**

This is the inflammation of the urethra or what is generally referred to as the slim tube. The male urethra helps to transport urine and the semen through the tract and out the penis. This inflammation causes itching, painful urination and swelling around the penis. All of these symptoms contribute to premature ejaculation as the penis is no longer in a perfectly functioning state.

## Excessive Alcohol Intake

The excessive intake of alcohol is known to be one of the most potent causes of erectile dysfunction, so it should not be completely bizarre that it also causes premature ejaculation. Too much alcohol in the body is responsible for what is medically known as 'Brewer's "Droop,' a state which affects sexual performance and is equally responsible for premature ejaculation. Countless cases have been recorded in which alcoholics could not at all gain erections.

When an erection is managed to be gained, the penis is not able to sustain the hard-on and has no choice but to give in to quick ejaculation in order for the muscles to relax and make the organ return to normal.

**Drug Use**

Some men have been exposed to some drugs that make them last longer in bed, and there have been testimonies. But not all of these drugs are genuine. Some of them, under some factorial irregularities present in the human body, start to work in reverse. Drugs are very potent substances that when used in the wrong way, can cause a lot of damage in the human system. Also, there are some drugs whose worst side effects result in premature ejaculation. If a man uses a class of drugs called opioids, then there is a high chance that sexual performance is lessened.

The opioid family of drugs is a category which was developed to serve as painkillers, including morphine, tramadol, and methadone. These drugs are highly effective, but they tamper with men's sexual system and organs.

Such drugs can cause an erectile dysfunction and a premature ejaculation.

## Laziness

At first, this might seem vague, and even funny, but the truth remains evident: we have lazy men in the world. Not to refer to them as weak, but we already know what the point is exactly. Some men do not have the right amount of strength to have sex for a reasonable time measure.

Due to so many reasons, these men have been found to ejaculate after three to five thrusts in and out of the vagina. Some do not have the strength to thrust well and having organs just as lethargic, they develop weak erections and expel semen all too soon during sexual intercourse.

## Stress

In some cases, stress and laziness are made to be synonymous causes. But that a man is stressed out does not mean he is lazy. Men who perform tasking or odd jobs all day long or men who work stretches of hours sitting on a chair are the ones that will be stressed out more at the end of the day.

When stressed, the entire body is weak and cannot function normally, as it did before.

When stressed men engage in sex, they often do not enjoy it. An erectile dysfunction may be caused, and then premature ejaculation kicks in. It should be noted that when the human system undergoes stress, it also affects him psychologically, making him want to simply ejaculate fast and get to rest.

## Psychological Factors

Having looked at the physical or medical causes of premature ejaculation, which is but one side of the two-sided coin, a flip is no doubt in order. However, it is imperative that one knows that the just explained causes can also be biological, just as it is medical. Given that a man's physical health has a lot of ways it affects his sexual performance, it will also give an idea that his psychological health can also have a hand in it. The psychological causes of premature ejaculation are fewer than the physical or medical or biological. But that does not in any way make them less factorial and potent.

Many people have the belief that the problem is caused by anxiety, frustration and lack of self-confidence. These are quite true, but in fact, they are mostly the results of premature ejaculation. However, these said causes may develop in the long term cases, often due to the fact that the man becomes stuck in an endless repeating circle of anxiety, ejaculation problems, frustration, and guilt. The common psychological factors of premature ejaculation include strict upbringing, sexual inexperience, early conditioning, traumatic background, stress, depression, teenage masturbatory practices, unresolved relationship, conflicts, and fear.

## Strict Upbringing

In society, there is a norm that convinces not only young males but females and adult as well that sex is a shameful, dirty, sinful and risky act. Many are also made to believe that sex should not be had except for religious purposes such as procreation; the making of babies. They are also told that sex should only be had in a very enclosed and defined matrimonial setting where a husband and a wife come together to pleasure themselves, bond and have children.

As such, these sets of people grow up with the notion that sex, if not had under these conditions, is an abominable, unclean and punishable act that can lead to the contacting of not just sexually transmitted diseases, but also as they are told, the bad and ugly traits as well as odd spiritual infections of the sex partner. Sex is then seen as a malignant act that can bring shame to one's family, especially in cases where it culminates into an unwanted pregnancy.

Young males in such societies, having been brought up in such a way, develop a notion of sex, which makes them fear and dread it. This is often a feature of premature ejaculation in teenagers who have been brought up in such a way, as they would want to quickly have sex and be done with it in order not to be discovered, infected or implicated. This is the effect that strict upbringing has on males that develop the premature ejaculatory tendencies.

## Sexual Inexperience

Lacking sexual experience is often viewed as a thing of shame and weakness in the world of men.

Younger men especially, go through phases of premature ejaculation because they lack orientation on the pros and cons of how to have long lasting and enjoyable sex. Many young men place great emphasis on potency and sexual performance and are often very keen to assert and prove their virility.

The sole reason for this is sexual inexperience. They do not know what to do and how to go about doing it. For example, some may not know that the strong will to assert their virility will lead to them ejaculating prematurely.

## Early Conditioning

A man's first sexual experiences have a way of affecting the later behavior of the same sex. Therefore, if the man has had records or irregular sexual practices, there is a chance that it will affect his future behavior. For example, if at a time in life, a man ejaculates rapidly in order to escape being discovered masturbating behind closed doors, or having sex, there are effects.

A man rushing the sexual act in such a way; in order to achieve sexual climax, has a lot of adverse effects it will cause later on, of which premature ejaculation is the most prominent. It results in the man unknowingly continuing to behave this way; ejaculating rapidly.

Once this behavior has been established, it is very difficult to break the habit. Additionally, cases have been found in which the behavior is genetic; a father with the behavior may genetically transfer it to his male child, although this is very rare.

**Traumatic Background**

Traumatic experiences previously in one's early life can cause sexual problems, as well as premature ejaculation. It may make the problems permanent and also cause a socially inappropriate behavior.

When a man is traumatically disturbed, probably due to negative sexual experiences, he may lack control over ejaculation. Sexually related traumatic experiences can range from being caught in the act of masturbation to being discovered while having sex, or being sexually abused as a child, adolescent or teenager. The chances are that the trauma could actually have been caused due to incidences of male rape. When men have these disturbances from the past, they can as a result of them have premature ejaculation problems.

## Depression

Depression, which is medically regarded as an illness, affects about 2 out of ten people and is a serious, long term and adverse condition. Its symptoms range from mood swings, down feelings, disturbed sleep patterns, low morale, and reduced sex drive.

Persons who are depressed often lose interest in sex and the symptoms of the illness affects their libido and their inability to get and sustain an erection. So, when this set of people disinterestedly engage in sex with their mood issues on, they experience premature ejaculation. Often, most depressed people, being aware of this, do not like to have any sexual relationship with anyone, and equally will shy away from sexual intercourse. Some of them are pretty dogmatic about it because it makes them angry and enraged.

## Performance Anxiety

This usually occurs with men that have either not had sex at all or haven't had it in a long time. Anxiety or pre-excitement of sexual intercourse often leads to them ejaculating all too early. This is mostly associated with men of younger ages, often found to be freaked out or psyched about sex, and wanting to have it at all costs.

## Teenage Masturbatory Practices

In cases where men train in such conditions and train themselves to ejaculate quickly to avoid getting caught in the act of masturbation, the habit often stays with them for ripe old ages in which the premature ejaculation problem is posed.

The habit becomes very hard to break once they become sexually active. One Airwick Van made a publication on social media about his problems with ejaculation, testifying peculiarly that he experienced a lot of trauma in his marriage because he virtually lived all through his bachelor life masturbating. According to him, it caused distress to both him and his wife, until he started taking suitable psychological remedies to the problem.

## Unresolved Relationship Conflicts

When there are series of disagreements, fights, quarrels, and turmoil in the relationship. There is bound to be discomfort, depression, and sadness, which often makes the man prone to not being able to have the suitable sexual performance level. In many cases, an unhappy man would want to condition himself to have sex quickly and get over with it. Also, a man could be affected by guilt, especially in cases where there a lot of secrets being hidden, probably the ones that have to do with the man cheating on his partner.

Similarly, a man would feel sexually inferior when he finds out his partner has sexual relationships with other people, making them always having it in mind that it is a result of their inability to satisfy their partners that led to it.

Factually every man has his bad days, and on such days anything could be the reason for his inability to last longer and/or satisfy his partner. This often leads to a lot of consequences. Premature ejaculation often culminates in broken relationships and marriages, because women, having sexual needs that need to be satisfied may prefer to move on to greener pastures to get their sex lives more interesting and a lot intensifying.

This causes distress in men, making them recline to themselves and decide not to go into any other commitment with a partner for fear of being discovered and then broken all over. On the side of the women, some wives who share their husbands' plight experience distress as well. In the long run, both parties are affected, and the effect may rub off on the other aspects of their lives such as social, corporate, religious, family and financial among others.

Premature ejaculation, having caused these problems and a lot of others, needs to be solved. All that is needed is a perfect orientation on how to curb the ramp of the seeming menace.

# CHAPTER FOUR

## Home Remedies for Premature Ejaculation

As there are physical/medical and psychological causes of premature ejaculation, there are also suitable remedies for them with respect to those causes. There are remedies men can devise and use at home, and then there are medical (drugs) as well as psychological ways to also solve the dysfunction.

### Home Remedies

There are countless ways of solving premature ejaculation at home, and most of them are usually done using natural ingredients such as fruits, oil, etc. It is often referred to be "how to cure premature ejaculation the organic way."

### *Watermelon*

This particular fruit has gone by many names. People have called it a natural Viagra. A watermelon relaxes blood vessels, without leaving any side effects. A man is advised to cut the watermelon into small pieces and sprinkle some powdered ginger and salt on them. Then, the dish is ready for eating. It can also be added to any fruit salad meal.

What is present in that recipe that does the trick is the phytonutrient known as citrulline, which increases the libido of the man.

### *Seeds of Green Onion*

The seeds of the green onions bulbs have been found to possess the perfect aphrodisiac qualities potent enough to help with the problem. The seeds can best be gotten at the early stages of the vegetable's life cycle. To come up with the natural remedy, clean the external leaf tops and take of the already decaying green parts, peel off the outer surface till you get a fresh, crisp onion, and then cut them into pieces to be eaten in recipes or in dishes. Alternatively, the seeds can be crushed and poured into a five teaspoon measure of water.

Afterwards, the powder is left to soak for about three hours, and the mixture can be taken before eating a meal. In the onions is present an antioxidant that has anti-inflammatory and anti-histamine properties, also having a chromium mineral that helps the body in the storage of nutrients, management of glucose and metabolic processes.

The potassium and Vitamin C components in the onions help to regulate the heart, enhance the number of sperm cells and circulates blood enough for a healthy sexual intercourse, with this, relieving men from premature ejaculation. Patients with heartburn and gastric reflux disease are advised to stay away from this remedy.

### *Ashwagandha*

This herb helps to enhance the strength of organs, boost their functioning and also help the entire body system to acquire stamina. The herb is known to help cure infertility, impotence, and problems in male libido, and also lessens negative feelings such as anxiety, stress, depression, insomnia, and sadness. By mixing one teaspoon of Ashwagandha root with one teaspoon of honey and one glass of milk, and consuming the glass on regular basis, one would be giving one's body the necessary components good for the nervous system and for the improvement of the flow of blood in the male genital organs, helping the man to achieve longer duration during sexual intercourse, hereby, relieving the man from premature ejaculation.

### *Ginger and Honey*

Ginger has aphrodisiac properties that help cure sexually related problems. Combining it with honey increases libido, performance and lustful feelings. To remedy premature ejaculation, grate a tablespoon of ginger and mix it with some amount of honey. Consuming the mixture every day in a month will make a man feel the difference. The recipe has anti-inflammatory and antioxidant properties that aid blood circulation, detoxification, and cure erectile dysfunction. This recipe is not good for men with diabetes, kidney stone and allergy for pollen and celery.

### *Asparagus and Mil*

Asparagus is a lily with medicinal properties. To get the recipe, take two teaspoons of Indian Asparagus (fine powder) and one glass full of milk, cover the lid and let it boil for 15 minutes, and strain the mixture and drink it thrice daily. Vitamins A, B3, and C are present in the mix, which works together to increase blood flow, increase sperm count and blood flow to the penis, enabling the man to delay ejaculation.

The combination of asparagus and milk have been found to be one of the most effective remedies for the premature ejaculation problem. Patients with low metabolism, allergy for leeks, onions, and milk should not use this remedy.

***Saffron, Almonds, Ginger, and Cardamom***

To get the recipe, soak ten almonds overnight in water, and peel off the skin on the next day. Blend the almonds in an electric blender with one cup of hot cow milk.

Add a little saffron, ginger, and cardamom to the mixture and drink it every morning. Zinc, phosphorus, manganese, iron, selenium, sodium, Vitamins A, B1 B2 B6 and E, copper, curcumin, caffeic acid, capsaicin, and magnesium are all present in the recipe, and these collectively help to control heart rate, blood pressure, promote red blood cells, release of energy and boosting of the sex drive. All these put together help men last longer in bed.

### *Cinnamon*

Very few people are aware of the fact that cinnamon bark can cure menstrual cramps, common cold, diarrhea, and premature ejaculation. For the men problem and to remedy it, take two teaspoons of organic cinnamon powder and mix it with five tablespoons of water. The mixture should be consumed twice daily after each meal.

The medicinal components of the cinnamon bark have a lot of ways in which it reduces flatulence. It enhances the flow of blood, making metabolism stimulated and boosted. The astringent properties are linked to medicinal components known as tannins, which also help in the prevention of diarrhea.

This remedy helps better if the man's premature ejaculation problem is caused by irregularities of impediments in the normalcy of digestion. Men that have diabetes or about to undergo surgery (usually in two weeks before) are advised not to use the recipe.

### *Banana*

This fruit has a lot of myths surrounding it. One accounts that the male organs of our ancestors, the ones that looked or had the shape of bananas were the one whose owners were able to enjoy sex for an extended period of time without having to worry about premature ejaculation. Well, no one can really attest to how true the story is, but what is paramount is that we draw a lesson or two from it. In the present day, and of a more provable matter of fact, bananas are good for enhancing libido and sex drive.

Sexologists prescribe that both men and women should consume at least five bunches of bananas a week to improve their sexual performance. Alternatively, a man challenged with premature ejaculation can blend bananas with other fruits to make a smoothie, or blend bananas alone and drink at least twice a day.

The iron and vitamin component in bananas help to boost blood circulation, aid digestion, enhance immunity to illnesses and assist hormonal balances.

It has been observed that men who crave banana and have it as their best fruit hardly have problems with lasting long bed, and in the same vain satisfying themselves and their sexual partners. The banana recipe is open to all and sundry, as it has no side effects and exceptional cases.

### *Garlic*

This is a natural medicine that helps increase blood flow to the penis and also helps to heat up the body. Garlic can be sorted in the low-flame using cow's ghee until its color turns golden. Take this every day or just chew three cloves of garlic to treat not just premature ejaculation, but erectile dysfunction inclusive.

### Eggs and Carrots

Egg and carrot when combined form a very potent remedy when mixed with honey. It helps to enhance adequate blood flow throughout all the organs, including the penis, and also helps the body reduce stress and anxiety. To come up with the remedy, take a half-boiled egg, slice them into bits and mix the pieces with some chopped carrots.

Adding four teaspoons of honey, blend the mixture into a fine, smooth paste. Taking the mixture every day for about three months will yield an astounding result, treating premature ejaculation and other sexual anomalies.

### *5-Hydroxytryptophan (5-HTP)*

This supplementary remedy works by increasing a man's serotonin level, which in turn enables him to relax both mentally and physically, helping the penis to relax perfectly in readiness for sexual intercourse. Likely, it will stop premature ejaculation all of a sudden, but it will slow down the process to help you last longer. The dosage is around 600mgs per day, which will take about 7-10 days before taking full effect.

### Kava

This is typically a herb that works similarly with the 5-HTP. It helps relax the brain's neurotransmitters, relieving the excessive excitement, and slowing down the man's reactions to boost the level of sexual stimulation. Kava also aids blood flow into the penis, helping men to maintain a longer lasting erection, but without the overexcitement and over-stimulation. To have the best results, the man is advised to take 100-200mgs of kava extract about an hour before engaging in sexual intercourse. Mixing the kava extract with a dosage of 5-HTP also makes it more effective.

**There are ways, other than natural home remedies, to cure premature ejaculation that have to do with behavior and physical exercise. Below are some helpful tips.**

### *Kegel Exercise*

This exercise helps to strengthen the pubococcygeus (PC) muscle, which is the main controller of ejaculation. Kegels is done by squeezing the same muscle as you would to stop peeing midstream, and that happens to be the Pc muscle. Clench the muscle for 10 to 15 seconds then release for another 10 to 15 seconds.

Repeat this five times in a row for three times in a day, and it will strengthen your PC muscle, enabling you to have control over ejaculation. There is a need to be consistent with the exercise to get the best results.

### *Special Thick Condoms*

There are special condoms that help reduce overstimulation during sexual intercourse. Sex does not feel quite as good when using a condom, so when you want to last longer, use a thicker condom or one that is well coated with benzocaine, which is one of those numbing agents.

By doing this, the level of sensitivity will reduce and help you to last longer. The brands that make the best kinds of these special condoms are Trojan and Durex. The thicker the condom, the longer you can delay ejaculation.

### *Deep Breathing*

Back in the days of black and white, we were made to take deep breaths almost for everything, unaware that it was actually a therapy to help us get control over activities. Taking deep breaths before and during sexual intercourse is a simple and effective way of delaying ejaculation for every man. One deep breath increases the oxygen content of the blood and causes the brain to release mood stimulating chemicals called endorphins.

This creates a calming effect, and as we are told, the calmer and more relaxed a man is before sex, the more he stands a chance of lasting longer. Simply inhale through your nose and hold the breath for three to five seconds, or more, and exhale slowly, preferably through the mouth. Repeat the sequence until you feel completely relaxed and ready to go.

### *Healthy Eating*

Experts and researchers have realized that a certain percentage of men with premature ejaculation problems do not have healthy diets, as their body systems are not provided with the necessary nutrients that will make the organs to function better and enable them to have long lasting sexual intercourses. To be sexually healthy, it is imperative that one observes healthy diets, with meals containing very helpful nutrients in their right proportions. A meal is by far more nutritious is the one that contains all the classes of food, as they will help the reproductive system and others function properly. Have fruits regularly. Blend different fruits with various combinations to make a smoothie and drink at least once daily. Avoid canned food and go for more natural, homemade and refilling meals. Remember; healthy eating makes one stay healthy.

**Apart from natural fruits and physical remedies, there are also pills that can be bought in the market that help to cure premature ejaculation. Although some of them are quite expensive and have not really received substantial appraisals, their reviews look promising.**

Below are some of them:

1. Delay sex pills

2. Man XXL

3. Pro Solution Plus

4. Premature X

5. Stallion Power

6. L-Argine

7. St. John's Wort

8. Detain-X

9. Ejacutrol

10. DelayMaxx

11. RixerXL

12. Duramale

13. Dapoxetine

14.  Modafinil

15.  Silodosin

16.  Prosolutioon Plus

17.  Delay Pills

18.  Enlast

19.  VigRX Delay Spray

20.  Climax Control

21.  Julian's Rock Hard Cream

These drugs have dosages that come along with their packs, bottles or from the pharmacist's direction. Once you find the one that works for you, stick with it and enjoy and be proud of your sex life.

## Psychological Cures for Premature Ejaculation

Psychology and premature ejaculation are an intertwined duo. As there are psychological causes, so also are their psychological remedies. These remedies vary from person to person, and more importantly, the reasons for the anomaly in the first place. Stanley E. Althof, Ph.D., from the Center for Marital and Sexual Health of South Florida, has analyzed the strengths and limitations of different psychological intervention for premature ejaculation. In his view, psychotherapy alone is the best for men or couples where the problem is clearly psychological, as in cases where the problem is caused by anxiety, depression or fear. The most recent approaches to psychotherapeutic cures to premature ejaculation emphasize that men should learn to control by learning new techniques, gaining confidence, lessening anxiety and learning better communication.

There are different types of therapeutic cures for premature ejaculation, and before delving into the main course, it is necessary to go for a spin around these genres.

**Individual Psychotherapy:**

This is most applicable for men who are not in any relationships, in that it helps them to address the solution to the problem of not wanting to go into relationships because they do not want to be embarrassed.

However, should the man be in a relationship already, this kind of therapy is effective if the problem is rooted in childhood experiences or youthful trauma, or excessive fear or hostility to women. Individual psychotherapy may take an exploratory turn into the real underpinnings causal to the reluctance of men to enter into relationships. It can also be behavioral, and specific approaches can be gathered from it to control ejaculation in general, enhance the man's attention to arousal and to help curtail anxiety. This therapy suggests ways a man can solve premature ejaculation alongside solving his relationship problems.

## Couples' Therapy

This helps couples unite to find the cause of premature ejaculation on the part of the man; where couples are motivated to seek the treatment as well while exploring the various factors that may be at play. According to Jerry Kennard, couples' therapy can be either exploratory, looking into issues in the relationship that contribute to sexual issues and premature ejaculation, or it may take a behavioral form, examining specific techniques around ejaculatory control and arousal that are worked directly with the couple together. This is also called "sex therapy."

## Psychotherapy with Medication

This approach involves the combination of drugs with psychological therapies. According to Dr. Althof, this may offer the best of both worlds, as the effect of certain medications to delay ejaculation can help to build confidence before psychological therapies are used. As a matter of time, the man can learn how to overcome his fear for arousal, and be advised to attend to other sensations. And once this is achieved, they can be weaned off whatever medication completely.

As is evident, the master to the psychological treatment of premature ejaculation is therapy. The several therapeutic cures the anomaly and a larger number of them have high success rates, based on general observations. However, therapy is but a branch of the psychological cure.

## Cognitive Behavioral Therapy

This approach involves teaching the patients how to recognize the way in which the negative thought patterns can be effective to the problem of premature ejaculation. It also teaches them how to fight against these using positive affirmations and cognitive restructuring. Basically, the idea is to stop the patient from worrying sick about the prospect of premature ejaculation, and the chances that he will have the problem during sexual intercourses.

This is done because stressing about the prospect only does worse by drawing unneedful attention to it. The patient is taught how to have sex that involves maintaining a calm attitude, letting him focus primarily on the partner's satisfaction. By doing this, it is very possible for the man to get out of his own way, leading to the enjoying results that have been long sought for.

## Psychotherapy

As obvious, this is another form of therapy, but this in context has to do with the convictions of the man and how they go long ways to contribute to premature ejaculation. This therapy is closely linked and lead by the Freudian teachings, especially the psychodynamic theory.

It is believed herein that the sufferers of premature ejaculation may, as a matter of fact, possess unconsciously, hostility towards women. As a result, their premature ejaculation is a way of getting the feminine lot into episodes of frustration, while getting their own satisfaction in the long run. Therefore, to cure the problem, the approach teaches the men to learn to accept women as an important and non-harmful and compassionate gender of people, enabling them to discard the schemes that they plot against them.

Virtually, psychotherapist does all that is possible to reach the inner minds of the patients and fish out their deepest, worst and most intentional of secrets as to why premature ejaculation seems to ruin their present lives, as a result of the convictions and decisions they have made in time past.

## Sex Therapy

This approach is very practical. It combines the CBT type with sex advice, or what is colloquially referred to as the sex talk. During this approach, sex therapists have sessions with the affected men to help them identify the various signs that indicate that they about to climax, and then recommend for them the 'stop and start' method, in which they literally stop moving during sexual intercourse so they can have some relaxation. This method has had 98% success. However, women need constant thrusting into their vaginas in order to reach the most enjoyable of orgasms; it is often called continual stimulation. This has caused many speculations but have never decreased the rate of success.

Also, women have been found to nevertheless reach their climax even with the abrupt stops and starts they get from the males. Inclusive of this sex therapy is the therapists' directing of the patients to garner for desensitizing agents that numb the excessive sensations. And to strengthen to pubococcygeus muscle, the patients are told to exercise frequently to control ejaculation. According to Keith Hillman, generally, using the cognitive behavioral therapy or just self-help to try and remove the anxiety associated with premature ejaculation is the best strategy. According to him still, one of the best ways to do that is to eliminate some of the pressure by focusing more on foreplay and trying techniques like the tantric massage where orgasm is no longer the focus or the goal of sex. Tantric (tantra) massage is a type of massage that uses sexual energy to achieve a higher state of consciousness.

## Conversations

This is the relationship talk. It is used by couples who are faced with premature ejaculation problems to see how they can have conversations between themselves. This method sometimes helps, for couples who have the problem as a result of the man's feelings of inferiority, worry, uncertainty, etc. Most times, when there are unresolved conflicts in the relationship, it affects the man's level of performance and prevents him from lasting long.

However, most couples fail to realize this, attaching the problem to less prone causes, and even creating more conflicts. Most sex therapists advise their patients to go back home, create some quality alone time with their partners, and have real conversations that will help relive the man of all the worry. Most women that complain to their therapists about their partner's premature ejaculation, and how they are left unsatisfied after it, are advised to be more sensitive when talking about it with the men in context. They are told to make the men understand that they having the problem does not mean they are worthless or weak in the relationship.

Women are advised as a matter of priority, to talk with their husbands using empathetic methods to elevate the negative feelings they have lurking inside of them. When these relationship conflicts are resolved, they often will feel naturally happy after opening up to their spouses. The watchwords here are honesty and empathy. Premature ejaculation should never be a cause for quarrels and backbiting, as it will only make matters worse. An unrushed, meaningful and healthy conversation will help a lot.

### Regular Exercise

A large number of physicians have published books that enlighten the general public on the need for constant exercise, stating quite countless of times that it helps men to keep their reproductive systems alive, functional and reliable. Working out helps to burn out excessive fats, as a result of this reducing the sugar and cholesterol level in the body, which are the leading causes of diabetes.

Exercising helps men to attain sexual stamina that will help them enormously during sexual intercourse. Statistics have shown that eighty to ninety percent of men who suffer from premature ejaculation do not keep themselves fit.

There are a lot of gains you can get from hitting the gym twice or thrice a week, and going on hikes on some mornings and doing some pushups before going to bed and after waking up. It is all about physical fitness, and it helps you maintain rigidity in sexual activities. Working out also keeps you mentally fit. Medicine shows that some hormones and brain fluids are released during exercise, making the trainer to be able to make quick and smarter decisions. In order to have a sexually healthy life, you have to be mentally prepared and fit as well, because it is only an intelligent mind that can have control over his ejaculation during sexual intercourse.

Statistics have also shown that 98% of men who work out are sexually healthy, having no premature ejaculation problem to deal with. Psychotherapists at some points, having evened the odds as to the reason why their patients ejaculate prematurely, and finding not just trace, asks them to take up good and regular exercise. In most of the cases, if not all, providing the diagnosis of the doctor is accurate, the direction often turns out with some very marveling results. The men testify of a tremendous increase in their abilities to withstand and delay ejaculation, leading to much healthier sexual relationships with their spouses.

It doesn't break a bone or twitch a nerve to hit the gym. In fact, it increases lifespan and makes one less susceptible to certain diseases and infections. Living a healthy life by exercising on a consistent basis can even help one to develop total immunity to a particular illness or disability or problem, such as premature ejaculation. This makes all the problem go away and creates a fresh avenue for

happiness in one's sex life.

# CONCLUSION

Helping affected men cure premature ejaculation has not been an easy task for all the parties involved. Nevertheless, progress has been made and successes have been recorded in and out and all over. But to know the cause of a problem is the first solution, and following this line of logic, this book outlined the possible causes of premature ejaculation, stating that they could physical (biological/medical) or psychological.

The book took time to highlight some of the effects of these causes as well, ranging from distress, depression, withdrawal, frustration, lack of concentration, relationship conflicts and most of all, breakups and divorces. But, despite the number of seemingly conk causes that a problem might have, it does not translate to it not having a solution or cure.

And following this logic as well, the book identified and explained in detail the various cures for premature ejaculation, based on what caused it. These solutions ranged from natural recipes to diets, drugs, therapies, relationship actions, and exercise. It is important to know that the causes of premature ejaculation differ from man to man, so do the solutions to it. So, the rightest thing to do is to find a cure based on what caused the anomaly in the first place, don't go putting square pegs in round holes, and end up wasting time, energy and money on a remedy that will not work for you. If you need further clarifications, see a doctor or a therapist who will guide you in the right direction. Sort for professionals only, as it has been found that a lot of quacks are out there proffering baseless solutions and working based on a trial and error mechanism.

To help men remedy premature ejaculation, it is advised that the men first get to the root of the problem with or without help and seek out ways to solve it in time. As the saying goes "a stitch in time saves nine." Nursing and covering up a problem will only make it grow worse, and the worse it gets, the more the solving process becomes more cumbersome and tedious.

Try to discover the problem early enough, and upon this, also try even harder to solve it earlier, so it will not go the long way of causing more problems with you, your work, social life, relationship, and marriage. Most seemingly wrecked men we see today are not as they are because they have a problem, it is because they didn't want anyone to know, or because they did not attend to it early enough, leading them to graver crises that they cannot get out of easily.

Lastly, every man needs to understand that the larger percentage of the race have premature ejaculation problems. So, you are not alone. What will make you stand out is your ability to be open when necessary, attentive and sensitive to everything that has to do with the topic. It can be cured, and it will be cured.

# THE END

www.ingramcontent.com/pod-product-compliance
Lightning Source LLC
Chambersburg PA
CBHW061937270726
48660CB00011BB/1868